Restore Yourself

a journey in coming home

By Elizabeth D. Vartanian

**Please consult your physician before doing any asana/physical poses or pranayama. If any suggested movement or breath work causes dizziness or any other ill effect, stop immediately. Listening to your body and its reactions is an important part of the practice. **

This book is dedicated to my Sukha Yoga Austin family (y'all showed up for me and yourself. I love you all!) and my guys (I love you!). A huge thank you goes to Nancy Alder, thank you for always inspiring me to share my passion!

Introduction:
Why Restorative Yoga?

In our fast paced, modern world, we are often moving quickly from one project to the next and sometimes doing up to five things at one time, but what are we really doing?

Restorative yoga asks us to do just one thing: s-l-o-w down. This description might just sound difficult for you and at first, it will, because the action in restorative yoga is the action of just being present without any other place to go.

So what exactly is restorative yoga?

Restorative yoga is a practice that may have three to seven postures (or asanas) that are held for a long period of time, while being supported by pillows, blankets, and/or blocks. Restorative yoga is also a practice in mindfully breathing in and out to switch into our parasympathetic nervous system, or our "rest and digest" action. The opposite of "rest and digest" is the sympathetic nervous system which is often called "fight or flight." When our "fight or flight" runs too long, our bodies start to exhaust, we are unable to digest our food properly, and our sleep habits tend to be disrupted. These are just a few of the extremes that can happen when we do not allow our bodies to switch gears. When we slow down, our parasympathetic nervous system is active which then allows us to breathe a little more fully, let our hearts to beat a little slower, and a calmness to come over us. The parasympathetic nervous system can be turned on by consciously breathing slowly. This is why restorative yoga is so important.

I have been teaching restorative yoga exclusively for some time now and I love seeing people "flip the switch" in their bodies as they take up this practice. Many come to class over-stressed, over-thinking, and lacking the fullness often exuded by those who have a regular self-care routine. It may take time to get into the habits that restorative yoga can create, but the time committed is well worth it.

There are many tools that restorative yoga uses. The postures are a way to soften areas of tension in our bodies, allowing us awareness of what it feels like and where it exists. Not only can we soften the friction we feel in our bodies, we can soften the thoughts in our minds, particularly ones that are destructive to our bodies and our external lives. A lovely benefit of having a regular restorative yoga practice is that as we gain control of stepping away from our thoughts and as we begin to heal our bodies, we also have a space to listen to our hearts, souls, and get to know ourselves in a very beautiful way.

How often have we questioned, "what am I doing?" Or "how did I get here?" The answers to these questions can be difficult to find, but it does not take a detective to see our patterns, habits, and actions when we take a closer look. The problem is, we think we are too busy to slow down to take a look. Perhaps it is fear of seeing ourselves as imperfect or works in progress. I would like to let you know that we all feel this way AND that we are all works in progress. Perhaps it is a worry of being "selfish," but self-care is the exact opposite. Slowing down can help us be our best selves, which helps everyone.

For myself, I know that it often feels selfish to take "me time," but I am a better person for everyone when I do. I like to take the time each morning to check in and make sure I am operating from a full cup. A short meditation, a cup of coffee in the quiet darkness of morning, and a few slow movements to connect me to myself so that I can be more present in my day.

By starting to incorporate stillness in your days, you are inviting in your truth and presence. You are saying, "it is ok to not be perfect. I am human and I am love." Through learning to not get caught in the rabbit hole of your thoughts, you are taking control of what you think and making space for more creativity. And by committing yourself to peeling away the masks you wear for work or friends, you allow yourself to continually grow and see that changes as they come instead of changing and not knowing.

This book starts the process of bringing these practices or tools into your life. By starting a home practice with restorative yoga, you can begin to get to know yourself better as well as bring the yoga off the mat and into everyday life.

How does this book work?

This book is broken up into six sections:
- Center
- Soften
- Expand
- Open
- Rest/Reset
- Emerge

Each of these qualities can be felt in a great restorative yoga class. We want to come to class and get centered from or for our day, soften into our bodies and breaths to be present, expand beyond or unfurling our bodies to occupy space, become open to receive love and feel our emotions so they may pass, rest/reset so the junk that remains can leave and the love we called forth can stay. Lastly, we can emerge from the practice fresh and renewed.

We will begin to look at each one of these sensations through meditation, the creative process (writing or art), postures, and ways to create these feeling in our homes or kitchens. This book can be read straight through or you can pick a section that calls to you to start. There are spaces for you to write notes, draw, and add your own reflections. The activities can be done in 10-15 minutes or if you want to really explore, you can lose yourself, or rather, find yourself, in an hour or two of exploring. Whatever feels right for you is what you should do. This book is about you and beginning the journey to Restore Yourself.

A quick note about the postures, set a timer for 3-5 minutes for each pose and keep a notebook nearby. After experiencing each pose, jot down how long you held the pose and how it felt in your body. Some asanas will feel great and you will want to hold them long. Others it will feel like an hour instead of a few minutes. No matter what, keep your breathing slow and mindful. Be gentle with yourself. These practices will take time to get comfortable with yourself and being by yourself. Keep at it, restorative yoga is worth it!

Center

What does it mean to be "Centered"?

When we step into a yoga class, we are often filled with scattered thoughts or thoughts of the past and future. It can be challenging to be present when events from the day play over and over in our minds or the anticipation for what will happen tomorrow bogs down the mind preventing us to be in the here and now. Centered means situated in the center or having a specific subject as the focal point. The first, "situated in the center" is similar to the concept of being balanced or like bringing two halves equal to bring harmony. The second offers up the idea of a subject being a focal point or bringing our awareness onto just one thing. In our practice of yoga, we will essentially be combining these two definitions together. For our purpose and in our yoga practice, we use the word "center" to mean "to place ourselves in the center of the moment, bringing awareness to what actually is happening NOW, both to and around ourselves."

In a restorative practice, we shift into centered as class starts. It is the first action we take to get into our bodies. Shifting into a place of being centered can take a lot of work to be present and get clear. Starting from this place of self-awareness, allows a deeper connection to our breath, to our body, and to ourselves.

Center: The Feeling

So what does it feel like to be centered?

Take a deep breath in, exhale slowly.
Keep those same slow breaths going and close your eyes.
I will wait right here.
You show up for yourself when you are ready.

Centered is a sensation of balance and of focus. When you can bring your full attention and awareness to the task at hand or the present moment to enjoy. All too often, life feels rushed or like we need to be someplace else. When we feel centered, we are in the right place, better yet we recognize that we are where we are and that is alright.

The feeling of being centered of course, is not a permanent one, but a moment we can bask in. The more often we find ourselves in the sensation of being centered, the more likely we can get back to it. Our bodies and minds want to be in that place of balance and focus. Our hearts and souls want to feel connected and present.

Being centered feels to me like I have an idea of what my day holds, that I have made space and time for my family AND for myself, and that I am able to take part in activities that I love. Let's explore how it feels for you to be centered!

Meditation to Feel Centered

Find a comfortable seat.
Set a timer for 7 minutes.
Shrug your shoulders, open and close your mouth.
Inhale fully, exhale completely.
Rock side to side
Slowly still that movement until you have found centered.
Close your eyes.
Feel the space you are in.
Allow the mind to focus on the present.
On your slow breath.

Listen until the end on the ring of the timer.
Open your eyes.
Note how you feel.

NOTES

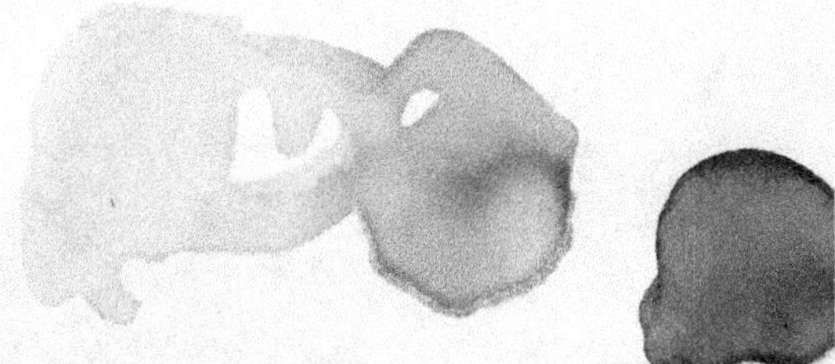

Creative Project:

What do you look like when you are centered?
Draw or write out how you feel and look when you are centered.
Include a list of things that help you feel centered.

Asana for Centering:

A folded blanket under head + a rolled up blanket under the low back. Two bolster/pillows under the calves. Arms wide.

Supported Savasana

Soles of feet together, knees wide.
A block under each thigh, knee,
or shin depending on
what feels supportive.
Press evenly through both sits bones.
Hands rest on thighs or knees.

Supported Baddha Konasana

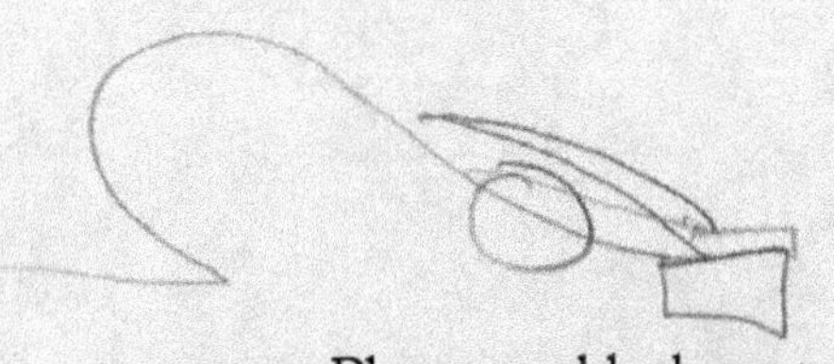

Supported Balasana with blocks

Place two blocks out in front.
Hips to heels, head to floor. Arms extend out, elbows on the blocks.
Bend the elbows, bring the hands to rest behind the head/neck.
Let the forehead/third eye connect to the floor.

Centered in the Home:

Make a shelf that holds photos, trinkets, or art that signify centered to you. Whether it be a family photo at the last reunion or you snap a selfie after doing the centered meditation, place a picture of you when you are beaming with the centered sensation. Trinkets from adventures where you felt balanced or from a time in your life you felt focused. Perhaps you have a place you love that invokes these feelings and you put a framed image of it up on your shelf. I have mine on top of my dresser, so that every day I start off reminding myself of this sensation.

After you have made your shelf, snap a photo and print out and add it to this page. Let it be ever changing. Swapping out pictures or trinkets as this feeling changes for you and placing photos of each shelf here to be a reminder.

Soften

Why soften in a world that asks us to harden?
We have this idea that is we were just a bit stronger or a little tougher life would not feel so hard. Is that really true though?

In our world today, we are quick to look at "soft" as weak or bad, but holding onto a firm outer edge or a ridge quality is like trying to eat uncooked spaghetti. It is a silly idea. Softening is not about being weak or being a doormat for anyone to wipe their feet on. It is about removing the hardness we accumulate in life through struggle, disappointment, hurt, and allowing space for us to see the joy and peace that already surrounds us. As the world becomes more isolating, more violent, more industrial, it becomes even more important for us to hold space for our potential to soften our minds and hearts to see the beauty that life around us holds. Beauty is everywhere, in all things.

Softening our edges, allows us to be mobile, flexible, fluid in our bodies, minds, and lives. Really asking ourselves to soften is another way of asking to let go of things, ideas, people and more that do not serve, help, or work anymore. We smooth the edges so that we can unclench, unwind, and yes, make space to breathe. All too often, we hold the hold breath when we feel pain, whether it be emotional or physical. As we use the idea of softening our hard edges, we will bring focus on the breath to let go.

Meditation for Softness:

Ganesh Mudra
This mudra (or hand gesture) cultivates the qualities of the deity
Ganesh who is the remover of obstacles.
As we meditate with this mudra, we are asking for softness in our
hearts and an ability to get through challenges.
Often asking for our own softness to see how we may create the
answers.
Set a timer for three minutes.
Place the left had in front of heart, palm facing outward
Thumb pointing down.
Place your right fingertips touching the left
The right palm faces toward the body, thumb up.
Roll the finger together, holding hands.
Seal the thumbs to enclose the grip.
Place in front of the heart.
Close the eyes.
Breathe slowly.
Soften the shoulders and the elbows, but remain firm in the hands.

Listen for the sound after the bell rings.
Release the hands.
Move slowly as you integrate back into your day.

NOTES

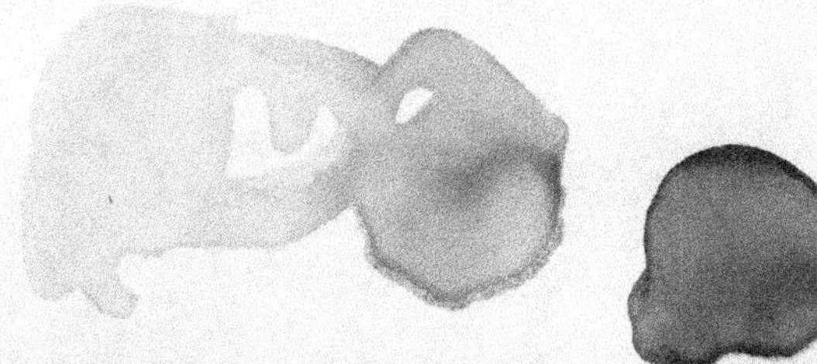

Creative Project:

Fill this space with how it feels when you soften your grip. When you let go of the word "should." Whether you write or paint or doodle, let this be a carefree space to create without any specific requirements.

Asana to Soften:

Lie on the back.
Bend the knees,
place the feet on the floor.
Put a bolster between
the knees and shins.
Drop the knees
over to the right.
Slide hips to the
left if needed.
Bring arms out to the sides.

Supta Matsyendrasana
Repeat dropping knees
to the left.

From all fours,
walk the hands away from the legs.
Keep hips over knees,
bringing
your heart + head
towards the floor.
Keep arms extended out.

Puppy Pose

Thread the Needle (arms)

From all fours,
slide the right arm under the left.
Placing shoulder on the floor.
Either extend the left hand or wrap around
the back towards the opposite hip.
Keeping hips over knees as best possible.
Repeating with the left arm under the right.

Soften in the Kitchen:

Making ghee.

Oh the slow melting of butter just oozes softness. The practice of making ghee or possibly what ghee is maybe foreign to you. Do not let that stop you from trying out this delightful (and simple) joy. Ghee is clarified butter, which means it is the process of separating out the milk proteins and leaving a liquid golden oil.

This recipe is simple, but still requires patience and awareness. Make it moving meditation and a practice in softening. I love taking the time to make this staple in our home. It asks me to be present as the making unfolds and it is fun to watch the transformation when softening happens.

What you will need:
- One pound of butter (16oz), preferably organic, grass fed, and unsalted.
- A medium sized sauce pan, a fine wire mesh strainer, cheese cloth, a spoon, a large measuring cup (at least 16oz), and a clean jar for storing.

Instructions:
1. Cut butter into cubes and then place in a sauce pan.
2. Using medium heat, melt butter. Then reduce down to a simmer.
3. Cook for about 10-15 minutes (depending on how hot your stove is). Over this time, the butter will go through several stages: foam, then bubbles, then seem to almost stop bubbling, then foam again. When the second foam happens, the ghee is done.
4. The melted butter should be a bright golden color and there should be reddish-brown pieces of milk solids at the bottom of the pan.
5. Let it cool slightly, 2-3 minutes before straining. To strain, line the wire mesh strainer with a few layers of cheesecloth and place over the large measuring cup. Discard the browned bits of milk protein.

6.   Transfer the golden liquid into the clean jar.

Ghee can last up to a month on the counter (at room temp) and longer in the fridge and can be used as an oil for cooking or melted on toast. Ghee has a stronger flavor, so a little can go a long way. Enjoy!

Expand

What does it mean to Expand?

Think about expanding like the morning stretch. We have been all curled up all night, maybe tense from dreams or sprawled out and relaxed, but we expand. We take up space. This is the sensation in our practice when we go beyond where we think our limit is, and maybe stretch just a millimeter more. We expand. We grow. Whether it be standing tall or lying on the ground taking up space, taking on a dream to make it come true, opening up the rib cage for more room in the heart, or trying out a new hobby, expanding is about going beyond any perceived boundaries.

Expanding is not striving or reaching, but truly taking up more room in this world. It is not goal oriented, but about moving in a slow manner that allows for growth but, not forcing. When we expand our bodies, our minds, and our hearts, we create room for more space, love, and joy.

Meditation to Expand Our Awareness:

Set a timer for seven minutes.
Lie down on the floor.
Take up as much space as feels comfortable.
Use props under the knees or head, as needed.
Take a full inhale in.
Exhale completely.
Close your eyes.
Focus on slowing the breath down.
Each inhalation expands the torso.
The ribs.
The belly.
Each exhale empties and softens.
Feeling the rise and fall of the breath.
Let the ocean like qualities of your breath fill your sense.
Each inhale the tide rises.
Each exhale, the tide releases.
Letting this wave like sensation wash over you.
Let that sensation of the wave of your breath radiate.
Towards your head.
Towards your toes.
Let the sensation of the wave of your breath radiate again.
From your body outward.
Feel it on your skin.
Feel the wave like motion moving the air that surrounds you.
Let the wave-like sensation surround you.
Listen for the end of the ring of the timer.
Slowly bring your awareness back the room.
Take in the sounds of the room.
Slowly begin to move the body.
Come upright.
Move slowly as you reintegrate back into your day.

NOTES

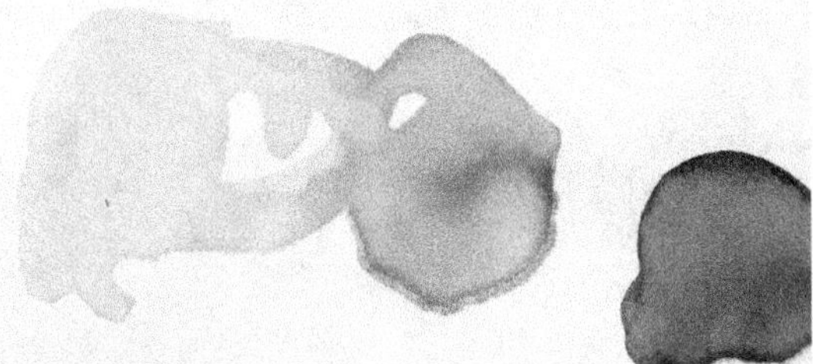

Creative Project:

Fill in things that are in your comfort zone and write down some things that are out of your comfort zone. Have some things that are out of your comfort zone that you want to try and circle them. This way you have a list of things to expand into doing.

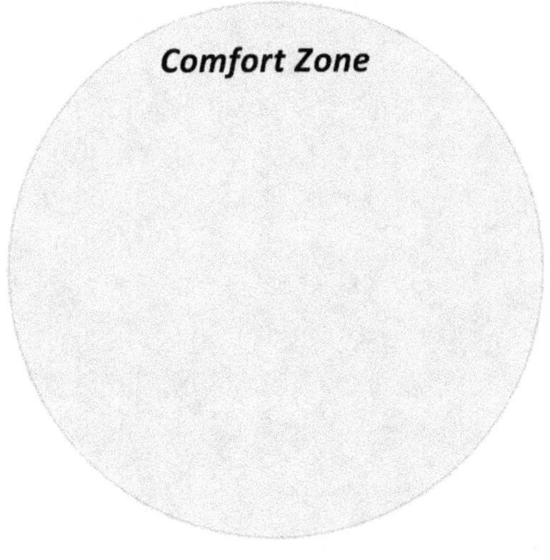

Asana to Expand:

With two bolsters/pillows
under the side belly
and lower ribs,
lie on the side.
Let top arm
stretch overhead.
Repeat on opposite side.

Side Body Opening

Balasana Variation

Hips to
heels head to floor,
walk hands over to the left.
Repeat on the right side.

Star Pose Variation

Lie on the floor,
arms and legs extended out. Use props as needed.

Expand in the Home:

Tackle a new project. Something small, like maybe putting up floating shelves in your room or painting a bold color on a wall you find drab. Step outside of your comfort zone, just a little and see what confidence it stirs when you succeed. Having a friend or family member as back up or around for support can be helpful in case you need another set of eyes or hands for the project.

Open

Why do we need to remain open?

Being open is not the same as letting everything in, it is not being without protection. When we allow ourselves to be open, to let go of the wall around the heart, the wall which is a boundary from the world, we are able to receive more love and joy. Openness is a two-way street, the world gets to see who we really are and we get to see the beauty in the world. Building a fortress around our love, who we really are, and locking ourselves away from life because it may be too intense is no way to live. Remaining open to new experiences, to allowing others to truly know us, and allowing ourselves to really know who we are, these are what we have been working towards.

We have drawn our awareness to be centered, we learned to soften the rigidness of our bodies and minds, we have expanded beyond our shrunken selves, we are ready to become open in our bodies, our hearts, our lives.

How to have boundaries AND remain open?

Openness does have its drawbacks. Asking ourselves to remain open when there is a chance of having our hearts broken, to be rejected, or worse not like who we see in the mirror, can be a challenge, but one well worth taking. We can remain open and have a limit to what we allow happen to us and to what experiences we seek. Being open does not mean you are a doormat for all those wanting to walk into the gallery of your heart. You can use caution, intuition, and common sense and still remain open.

When we have excess openness, we need to take a step back to set our space. Feeling too open can be a sense of vulnerability or over emotional including overly happy can be balanced out by taking child's pose or simply close your eyes. Inhale and set your space around you. Exhale and allow that space to be full of love and to remain open. Inhale and recite to yourself, "This is my space. Nothing may come through this space that I have not accepted." Exhale love.

Meditation for Remaining Open

Metta Meditation

Repeat each section three times, out loud.

May I be happy.
May I be healthy.
May I know peace.

(Choosing someone you know and love)
May you (insert name) be happy.
May you be healthy.
May you know peace.

(Choosing someone you have had a falling out with)
May you (insert name) be happy.
May you be healthy.
May you know peace.

(Choosing an acquaintance or mail person or someone you have
encountered in your day)
May you (insert name or how you know them) be happy.
May you be healthy.
May you know peace.

(Choosing to send love to all beings everywhere)
May we all be happy.
May we all be healthy.
May we all know peace.

NOTES

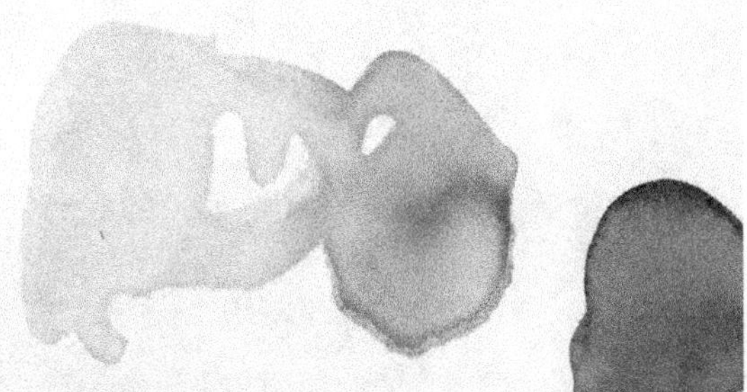

Creative Project:

What does being open look and feel like? Whether you write, paint, or doodle create something that shows you as being open. Open heart. Open mind. Living your best life.

Asana for Remaining Open:

Supported Matsyasana

Roll a blanket/towel into
a cylinder.
Place under
the spine from hips
to head.

Supported Baddha Konasana

Slide a bolster/pillow under the legs,
then put Soles of
feet together and let
the knees go wide.
Place two bolsters/pillows
behind the back
and rest down.

Openness in the Home:

Print photos of places you love, people you love, and photographs of yourself that you love. Find photos of places you want to visit or get some maps of cities you would like to explore. Have them framed or create a collage, but make sure you place them on a wall or shelf that you will see every day. Take time each day to remind yourself the importance of being open. Of coming from a place of love. Of being more you.

Rest/Reset

What does rest do for us?

What does it not do for us might be a better question! Resting is not only the most important thing we can do every day, but it is also the most important part of our yoga practice. Just like getting enough sleep allows for our bodies to repair themselves, some of our organs to have a break, and to generally refill our "tanks," at the end of our yoga practice we want all that we have done to settle into our bodies, minds, and hearts. We want to allow the things that we have let go of, whether they have been old thought patterns or tension in the shoulders, to dissolve and be fully released. Likewise, we want intentions that were set and things we brought into ourselves to remain. Our resting time is like hitting the reset button. It provides us with the ability to shift and get perspective.

Meditation for Rest:

Yoga Nidra

Lie on the floor or find a comfortable seat in a chair.
Get comfortable.
Take a moment or two to settle in.
Close your eyes.
Feel the fluidity of your breath.
You are safe.
No matter what your experience is today,
this practice is working.
Draw your awareness to your right foot, ankle.
Calf, shin, knee.
Notice your right thigh, your hips.
Draw your awareness to your left foot, ankle.
Calf, shin, knee.
Notice your left thigh, your hips.
Feel your spine, your belly, your ribs.
Your shoulders, your collarbones.
Notice your right hand, wrist, forearm.
Elbow, upper arm.
Notice the notch at the base of the throat.
Notice your left hand, wrist, forearm.
Elbow, upper arm.
Notice the notch at the base of the throat.
Feel the neck, the face, the ears.
Feel the crown of your head.
Become aware of the back body.
The front body. The midline.
Bring awareness back to the breath.
Slowly open the eyes and bring movement to the body.
Move slow as you integrate back into your day.

NOTES

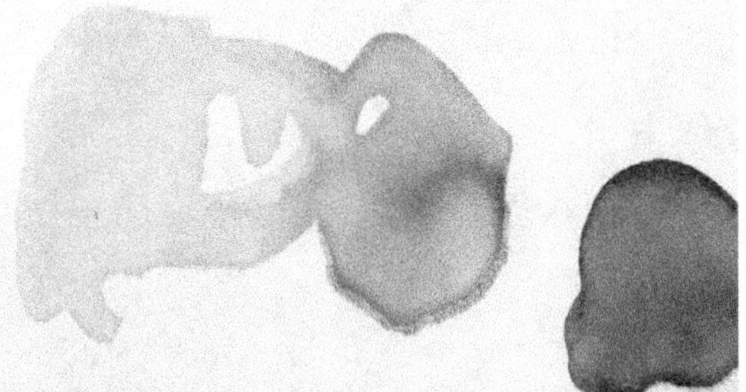

Creative Project:

Write or draw what it is to be rested. What does a reset look like for you?

Asana for Rest/Rest:

Legs up the Wall

Bring one hip close the wall
and swing legs up while the
back comes to the floor.
Place a bolster/pillow
under hips or
head depending on
what feels best.

Rest in the Kitchen:

Baking is a great way to experience rest/reset. Often times, recipes call for us to create and then let them "chill" making it a perfect reminder that everything needs a time out. Below is a recipe for bread (and gluten free one after that) that I often make for my family. There is something comforting to me about making bread, it takes a bit of intuition and a whole lot of awareness to make sure you get the dough right. Enjoy and when the dough is resting, take a few minutes to rest yourself too!

Basic Bread Recipe:

What you will need:
- 2 tsp dry yeast
- ½ cup lukewarm water
- 1 tbsp. honey or sugar
- 3 1/2 cups organic unbleached white flour
- 1 tsp salt
- ¾ cup cold water
- ¼ cup of olive oil
- A bread pan or baking sheet
- A mixing spoon, a wood cutting board or a Silpat

Instructions:
1. Combine the 2tsp of dry yeast, ½ cup of lukewarm water, and 1 tbsp of honey or sugar. Stir gently and let sit 15 minutes.
2. In another bowl, combine salt and flour.
3. Once the yeast, sugar/honey, and water combo has become bubbly, add the ¾ cup of cold water and the olive oil.
4. Make a well in the flour, salt combo and gently pour the yeast combo into the flour. Stir by hand until mostly combined. Then turn the dough onto a floured board or baking mat. Knead until dough is soft. The textures should be slightly sticky, but not overly wet.
5. Place the dough in a large bowl, cover well, and set the bowl some place warm. Let the dough rise for one hour.
6. Punch down the dough and knead a little, pulling in some air into the dough. Then place the dough in a greased bread pan (or

form into a round and place on a greased cookie sheet). Cover and let rest for another hour.

7. Heat oven to 400 degrees and after the dough has rested and risen, place in the oven.
8. Bake for 20-25 minutes depending on your oven. Keep a close eye on the bread as it bakes. Top should be golden brown.
9. Remove from oven and let cool before taking out of the bread pan or taking off the cookie sheet. Enjoy warm or share with a friend.

Basic Gluten-free Bread Recipe:

What you will need:
- 1 tsp dry yeast
- ¼ cup lukewarm water
- 2 tbsp. honey or sugar
- 3 1/2 cups gluten-free flour (I use Namaste foods brand, but you can also do 2 cups organic rice flour, ½ cup tapioca flour, ½ cup organic potato starch, ½ cup organic arrowroot powder, and 2 tbsp xanthan gum)
- 1 tsp salt
- 1 ½ cups of room temp plain almond milk
- 2 tbsp of olive oil
- 1 tbsp apple cider vinegar
- 3 room temp eggs
- A bread pan
- A mixing spoon, a wood cutting board or a Silpat

Instructions:
1. Combine yeast, honey/sugar, and warm water. Let sit for 10 minutes.
2. Mix almond milk, oil, and apple cider vinegar until combined. Add eggs, beating in one at a time. Add yeast mixture after it has sat.
3. Mix flour and salt together. Create a well and pour in yeast/milk combo. Mix well either stirring by hand or in a stand up mixer.
4. Pour into a greased bread pan and cover loosely with greased wax paper and then a towel. Let rest is a warm spot for up to an hour.
5. Pre-heat oven to 350 degrees. Remove towel and wax paper from the bread and cover loosely with foil to prevent over

browning. Bake for 25 minutes, then remove the foil and continue baking for another 30-40 minutes depending on your oven.

6. Remove from the oven and let cool completely before removing from pan.

7. Enjoy or share with a neighbor!

Emerge

When we leave the cocoon.

Post-practice bliss is a real thing, but what happens when we leave the cocoon of our practice to enter back into the world? When we first start practicing yoga we see the practice as separate from our "off the mat" time, slowly though there becomes a merging of the two. Life is the practice. Yoga is in all things.

Leaving the cocoon then becomes this moment after we emerge from our savasana (earned rest) and we begin to notice that in some way we have transformed. Something has changed. We might not be able to put a finger on it right away, we may not even notice it for months to come, but some part of us has changed. As we have made effort to consciously become more aware of who we are and what it is that we are carrying with us, parts of us has shed away as we embrace something new. We are always changing with each new experience we have and it is just a matter of being present enough to notice.

Meditation for Emerging:

Soham Meditation

This is variation based on the mantra soham, which is believed to mimic the sound our breath makes when we inhale and exhale. So-ham translate as "I am that" or "I am." We will use this phrase as a base.

Set a timer for three minutes. Close your eyes, place your left hand to your heart. Right hand out like you are taking an oath.

Inhale: I am

Exhale: (let whatever word comes fill the blank)

Repeat, each exhale becomes a new word. A role you play, an adjective that describes you. Let words that feel scary or too big come anyway. Let them be a coat too big for you to grow into.

After the bell rings, the last three exhales are: Inhale, I am… exhale, whole (you are already complete) Inhale, I am… exhale, strong (you carry the strength of 100 people, act like it) Inhale, I am… exhale, infinite (you are divine source, you are amazing!) Take a moment. Move slowly as you integrate back into your day.

NOTES

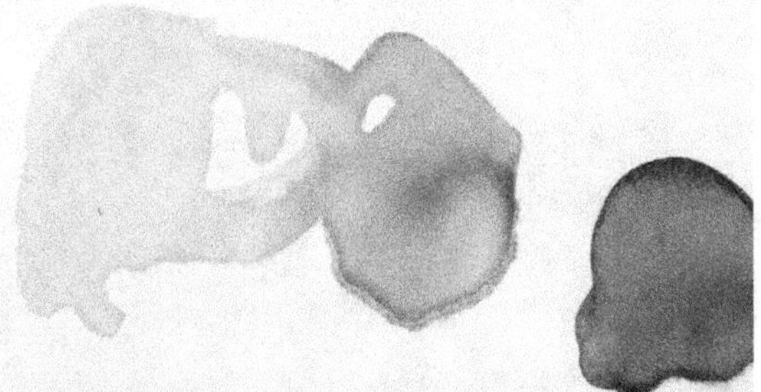

Create Project:

What does it feel like to be you? Draw or write out how you feel right now.

Asana to Emerge:

Inhale: tilt tailbone up,
let belly drop,
move the heart forward,
lift the head.
Exhale: tuck tail,
round spine,
draw chin to chest,
press through the hands.
Move with the breath
a few rounds.

Cat/Cow

Sukhasana,
sealing in class

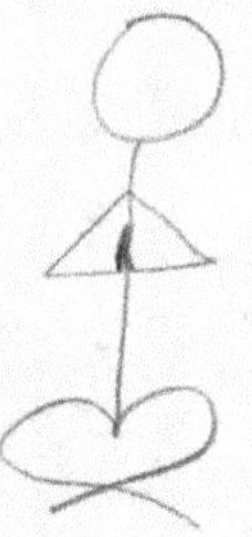

Take a comfortable seat.
Draw palms together at the
heart and close the eyes.
Give gratitude
for the practice.
Give thanks for all.

Emerge in the Home:

It is time to come out of your shell and there is no place better for this
to happen than in your home. Be a little more you than the day before.
Wear the dress you have been waiting saving for a special occasion.
Wear your hair the way you like it.
Go and do something adventurous.
Pretend you are having lunch in Italy if you are feeling the pull of
travel.
How can you be more you today? Start today (and every day) to
Emerge in your life.

Reflection on Restore Yourself:

Restorative yoga is a wonderful tool to come to know yourself and this book has many offering for you to choose from. Whether you open a random page and take practice or pull a posture from each section to make a peaceful home practice, the options are endless as to how you come home to you.

My Hope is that you start with what feels comfortable and that you end up doing it all, because as you feel and get to know yourself better, you trust the process and the practice.

I have added some extra pages at the end for notes on sequences you enjoy. Make your own little practices, take a pose from each section or pick three sensations you want to invoke. Create a home practice that suits your time frame, your needs. Add some meditation to your morning, while the coffee is brewing or waiting at a red light. You can record yourself reciting the meditations on your phone and play as necessary. Let these practices become your way of getting to know yourself. Allow them to be fun and inspiring. Most of all, I hope you learn to be comfortable with you.

Asana Sequence

Asana Sequence

Asana Sequence

Asana Sequence

Asana Sequence

Acknowledgements:
~~

There are so many people that had a helping hand in the making of this book. To my man Matt, you are my rock! Thank you for all the love and support. For supporting me as I take on the world to bring more love, light and yoga in the world. Even when you have no clue what I am talking about, you are always the first to lift me up. Thank you so much for that. I have to thank my friend Nancy Alder for inspiring me with this idea. I know you'll just say I took it and ran with it, but truly thank you!! Thank you for co-writing two books with me which gave me the confidence to do this.

To my community of restorative yoga peeps here in Austin, TX, this book is for you! Thank you for showing up to your practice and to yourself every week. Huge loves to my Sukha Yoga Tribe, specifically: Jacqueline St. Pierre for being an extra set of eyes, Erinn Lewis and Mark Heron for Sukha and the beautifulness you have created (and I get to be a part of), and a special thank you to Edna, woman, just thank you from the bottom of my heart. To my Once Over community, thank you for being my "first students" in the tree house, thank you for the amazing coffee and the great conversations. Melissa, mama, I could not imagine a better friend to have. I love our coffee dates and I do not know what I would do without getting to randomly text you! Thank you for being my tribe! To my teachers: Elena Brower (mama, goddess, thank you for listening, for your advice, and for your support!). Thank you to Kelly Morris for The Infinity Call, damn your meditations make me a better person.

To my family, thank you!!! I love you. Thanks for encouraging, teasing, hanging out and enjoying beers together. Family, I love you!! Mom, Pap, Carol, and Dad, thank you for always supporting me even if you are unsure. To my lady tribe: Rhokel Normington, Robin Chambers, and Karla DeLong, thank you! You are always in my heart and you will always be. To Bug and Bear, you both are my teachers, my heart and soul. I love you both to the moon and back. This book and so much of my yoga or writing is inspired by you both.

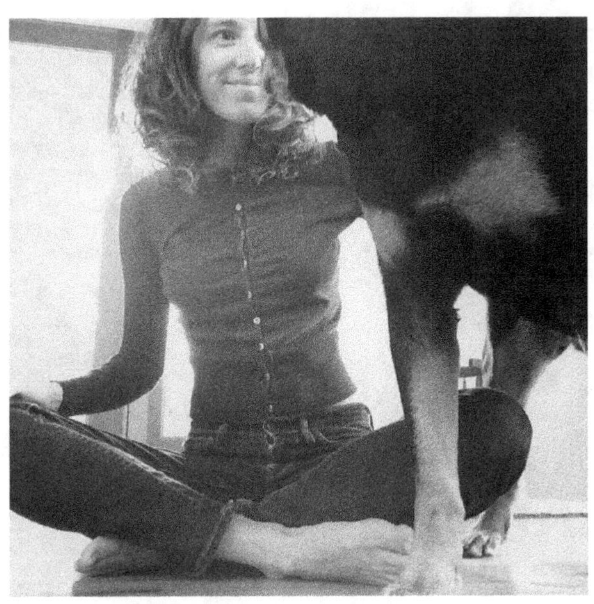

Elizabeth Vartanian is a yoga teacher, writer and mama in Austin, TX. Her carefully crafted classes include a loving blend of restorative and yin yoga, myofascial release, along with space to come "home" to your body. The soft surrender of restorative offer yogis a chance to leave class feeling energized and supported. Liz's classes feel like a community and students are often surprised with homemade goodies after long relaxing savasanas. Her training with viniyoga teachers during her 200-hr has offered her a chance to lead yoga practices with authenticity and heart but, from a place of safety and knowledge. Liz is a writer whose work was featured in OM Yoga Magazine. The delicate balance she strikes as a yoga teacher and mom was highlighted in Origin Magazine. She is the co-author of "The Living Mala" and "The Living Mantra." When not teaching yoga, Liz can be found with her family where there is coffee, good friends, toy trucks and a body of water!

www.ingramcontent.com/pod-product-compliance
Lightning Source LLC
Chambersburg PA
CBHW050929260726
48660CB00001B/471